D1433004

Now's the Time Self-Advocacy

Now's the Time
Self-Advocacy

and Your Breast Cancer Journey

JAG KAUR TAKHAR

This book is dedicated to my family, friends and all the communities.

Especially:

God – who has given me second chance to live and make this book happen.

My grand-parents Charan Singh and Mohinder Kaur (if I had to make one wish I want them to be my grandparents in every birth, gone too soon).

My parents Mohan Singh and Rajvir Kaur.

Jeevan and Shaan, my wonderful sons, who make me proud everyday.

My sisters – Raman, Raj and Manpreet who came to help me.

My cousin Nev, and her husband, Rashpal from Indianapolis.

All my friends from India, UK and Canada

To those who are currently need of some guidance – I hope you find it helpful. Now is the time for self-advocacy. To speak up and save lives.

I hope you can all speak up for yourselves to save family members, neighbours and friends.

Contents

- Preface -
Jag's Story

Breast cancer is a part of every woman's life, whether she has it or not. The fear, when touching your breast during self-examination. The knowledge of breast cancer in your family history. The waiting for results from a mammogram.

My story is about self-advocacy. My diagnosis didn't follow the standard route—discovering a lump through breast self-examination, or a doctor finding cancer through a screening. In these cases, treatment starts right away. I had to fight for my diagnosis. I found my own symptoms, but nothing was done when I reported them and asked for further investigation. It twisted things. I believe that if they had diagnosed me in June, when I had first reported symptoms, my breast could have been saved. If I hadn't learned to self-advocate, however, I could have lost my life.

∽

I've made a few international moves in my life, and a few interprovincial ones, too. I was a single mom, with two young boys. My husband died in early 2012, when my children were two and a half and seven. But I survived this huge loss. I thought I could handle anything. I was hardcore. And then, the long weekend of September 2017: my cancer diagnosis.

The journey wasn't easy. It was overloaded with pain, grief, depression, sleepless nights, and fear. My life was a constant stream of medical intervention, including drugs, needles, ultrasounds, X-rays, and CT scans. Then there were the terrifying side effects: hair loss, blistering skin, nausea, and pain.

Today, I am blessed to be a cancer survivor. The experience was both exhausting and exhilarating. Not just for me, but for anyone walking with me on this journey.

When I was diagnosed, I knew I was not alone in having to face cancer. Millions of warriors around the globe had struggled before me, and millions more continue to face cancer every moment of every day. So, I was not alone. I promise you: you are not alone either.

Breast cancer awareness is essential. It can lead to early detection, which saves lives. It may seem that we are inundated with awareness campaigns, screening tests, fundraisers. But for minorities, where there are language barriers and cultural gaps, these are still not enough. In Indian culture, for example, cancer is not discussed. It's a matter of family honour.

Anyone who has been dealt the bad hand of cancer understands that no amount of empathy or sympathy will end the psychological struggles of diagnosis and treatment. There's no magic pill to take that allows you to overcome the internal chaos you'll experience.

I am a living example, and I urge you: don't live in fear that cancer will kill you. One way or another, we all die. It's universal law: one who is born must face demise. Why live in constant fear?

Fear is a hurdle in the way of healing. Once you know this, and find your spirit, you'll have nothing but clarity. Remember: everything is temporary.

I admit, I was bitter about cancer at first. But I soon became determined to enjoy every moment of my life while suffering its side effects. Cancer left me the same way it entered. Now,

I think of it as a break from my busy life and responsibilities. Getting seriously ill makes us realize how beautiful life is, in simple terms. We don't need too much to be happy. Life is about making the most of what you have in the present, not what you are going to have in the future.

I'm not a celebrity, tycoon, or doctor. This is not a medical textbook.

This is a chronicle of my journey. It's meant to assist those who need it, whether they are a patient, survivor, or caregiver. It's meant as a guide along the way, so you can be prepared. I hope that reading this book will give you courage, instilling both knowledge and awareness. I've tried to describe my experiences as I went through different procedures and treatments. Where applicable, I've added detailed information I've gathered on how, why, and when these processes are carried out, as well as what to expect as a patient.

I want to dedicate this book to each person who struggles to find information when they, or someone they love, is hit by cancer.

This is my journey.

What is life?
A breath in a moment.
- **Jag Takhar**

- Chapter 1 -
Diagnosis

Summer 2017 was proving to be a hot one.

Everything was going smoothly, though. I couldn't complain. My kids were growing up well. I lived the typical life of a realtor: chasing clients and hosting open houses on weekends.

I also enjoyed some time with a friend who was visiting from England. She stayed with me for a day or so, and we went to shopping malls and the beach with my kids.

While shopping, I found a lovely evening dress to wear

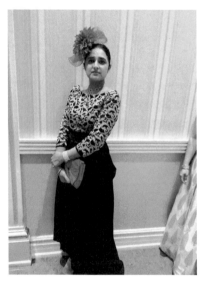

at an upcoming wedding reception. I kept it in my closet for weeks and was so excited to put it on. It was going to be a big, fat wedding, and I wanted to stand out from the crowd in style. I had a pair of red sandals and a red clutch from Marks & Spencer, but I still needed a statement piece: jewelry or a hair fastener. I ended up creating something quite stylish myself. I bought a hairband with a net from Michaels and added a flower to it. Very stylish indeed!

One hot day in May, after taking a cool shower, I noticed my left nipple was a little dry. I didn't think much of it. I thought it might be due to the weather, or the padded bra I wore.

On June 4th a friend of mine from college joined me for the Teeyan da Mela festival in Brantford. We hadn't seen each other in 17 years! It was so lovely to spend time with her. We were close, and I felt comfortable enough to tell her about my nipple soreness. She suggested I see a doctor.

I was already seeing a physician about my heavy periods so at my next appointment I mentioned my nipple. The physician explained they could only address one ailment per appointment, and that I would need to make another appointment to discuss my concerns. In the meantime, I had an appointment to see a gynecologist about my heavy periods and low iron.

Several weeks passed. It was July 30th, the day of the big wedding reception, time to put on my stylish dress. I needed to put stickers over my nipples—this was a deep-neck dress that didn't really suit a bra—but my left nipple had become wet and was peeling; the sticker was painful. When I came back from the party that night, I gave myself a breast exam.

I started to worry.

Another few weeks passed. My left nipple was still sore. Then it started leaking milk. There was no chance of my being pregnant. I had been single for over five years.

After another few weeks, pus started coming out of the nipple.

I Googled the symptoms and was deeply concerned by what I found.

It was hard to get an appointment with my family physician, so I went to see his partner. I told him I had a nipple infection—that pus was coming out. Instead of doing his due diligence and giving me a physical examination, this doctor simply prescribed me some antiseptic cream.

On August 4th I saw the gynecologist, who prescribed me birth-control pills as a means of regulating my menstrual flow. For some reason—perhaps a gift from God—I didn't get around to filling that prescription. I was later told that these birth-control pills could have encouraged the cancer to spread.

At the end of August I was taking my aunt and uncle to Vaughan, so my uncle could meet with his specialist. They needed a ride and someone who spoke English to translate for them. On the way back, I told my aunt about my nipple.

"We can't take any more bad news in this family," she said, referring to my nephew who had recently died. He was only 29 years old and had just finished his residency in Los Angeles.

As soon as we got back from Vaughan, I went to a walk-in appointment at my family physician's clinic in Brampton, and insisted the doctor perform a physical.

I was put in an examination room and the doctor came in with a female nurse who would be present while he examined me. Sure enough, he found a lump in my left breast and gave me a referral letter to get an ultrasound at the nearest lab. I called the lab and booked an appointment the following day.

Ultrasound

As many women who have been pregnant know, ultrasound is a way to take pictures of the inside your body using high frequency sound waves that you cannot hear. It's different than an X-ray because it doesn't use radiation and can take pictures of tissues, like organs, fat, and muscle. An ultrasound can be used to detect tumours.

What to expect:

For a breast ultrasound there is no preparation. Just remember not to apply any lotions or powders to your breasts. For other ultrasounds, such as renal, abdominal, or pelvic, you'll be given preparation instructions.

When you go in for an ultrasound, you'll be taken to a changeroom and given a gown to change into. It's a good idea to wear a two-piece outfit (not a one-piece pantsuit or dress), so you don't have to be completely naked under the gown. For a breast ultrasound, you'll need to remove your bra as well as your shirt. You must wait in the changeroom until you're called to the ultrasound room.

For the ultrasound, you lie on a table. The technician confirms who you are by asking your date of birth and/or other personal details. Then, they move a wand, covered with a clear gel, over your skin on the area where the pictures are to be taken. Sometimes you'll be asked to hold your breath for a couple of seconds and they will also move you in different positions so they can get images at different angles.

When they're done, you'll be given a towel to wipe the gel off, and then you'll be taken back to the changeroom to get dressed.

Results can take anywhere from one to 72 hours, depending on the facility and the urgency of the exam.

At the ultrasound, the sonographer didn't say much. Instead, she studied my face. Every time she measured a red dot, I got more suspicious. I had been trying to stay positive but my energy was dwindling.

The next day, a Friday, the doctor called me to his office to discuss the results. I went in, still trying to be positive, and saw him standing in the corridor. His face was hanging.

"Why do you look so down?" I asked casually.

As we settled into the examination room, he gave me the news. "You have breast cancer, and it has spread."

I was shattered. I literally screamed. I pictured my kids' faces and wondered who the hell was going to look after them.

When I asked him how much it had spread, he said he didn't know yet. We needed to do further investigation.

I was left thinking the worst.

It all seemed so unfair. For the past two months I had a leaky nipple and, prior to this, I had been feeling fatigued.

A year and a half before my diagnosis I asked my doctor to send me for a mammogram. He denied my request.

Now, this guy tells me I have cancer—and it has spread.

How can a family physician be so lazy and careless in diagnosing this dreadful disease? Nipple discharge is the first symptom of ductal cancer, and my doctor missed it. His thoughtlessness put my life at risk.

The picture below shows my family physician's notes. It's proof I told him I was worried about cancer. Look at what he wrote: of course I was "concerned" stupid! It wasn't just a "possibility," was it? It turned out to be my reality. I was so angry. I felt like my family physician and his partner had fucked up my life. I was devasted, and also wanted to kick their asses.

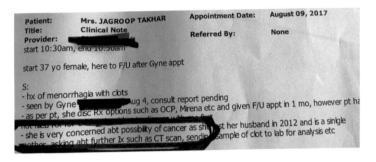

Next week was the Labour Day long weekend. It was horrible, even worse than the week before. I went from being normal and healthy to someone with breast cancer. Of course, I couldn't get a hospital appointment until the weekend was over. Believe me: getting diagnosed on the evening of a long weekend is not fun. My doctor's staff assured me they had booked a mammogram at Credit Valley Hospital on Tuesday, the first business day after my diagnosis.

I couldn't stop obsessing. How can doctors be so negligent? Did mine assume that at 37 I was too young to have cancer?

All I could think about was death and caskets. Imagine being a single mother of two, with no immediate family in Canada, somehow managing to have raised your kids on your own for five years, and then finding out you have cancer. Every second of my days was filled with sadness. I couldn't breathe.

What is life? I wondered.
Just a breath in a moment, and nothing more?

Breaking the news to my family was another challenge. Most people assume the worst—death—when they hear "cancer." Whom would I tell? My mom wouldn't be able to take it. I eventually told my brother-in-law, but I swore him to secrecy. I wasn't ready for my sister to know yet.

I was bombarded with negative thoughts, just like in 2012 when my husband passed away. I decided I should never have left the UK. Canada had wrecked my life twice. Stranded in North America, I felt alone, frustrated, helpless, and vulnerable.

I decided the person who would best understand what I was going through was someone who had gone through the same thing: my friend whom I will call Sam. Sam was still going through cancer treatment and was very sympathetic. Sam and his wife, whom I will call Dee, came to see me on the Monday of that very long weekend. Dee brought me samples of wheatgrass juice, soursop leaves, Indian basil, and moringa leaves: these are thought to detoxify the system. We talked about how Sam managed his cancer. Dee had more to tell; she was the one who worked, took care of the house and the finances, and dealt with the kids, on top of caring for her husband.

- Chapter 2 -
Breast cancer basics

Cancer is a group of abnormal cells, not killed by the body's immune system, that multiply rapidly. Those cells travel through the bloodstream and can spread throughout the body.

The body makes new cells that start out in an immature state and change into a mature state. Mature cells become working cells and these are what run our system. When these cells get old or if they are abnormal, they die. That's the way things are supposed to go. Cancer happens when something goes wrong with this process. The body keeps making cells, but the old or abnormal ones don't die; they just get in the way of the normal cells. That's when people get sick—when the normal cells can't do their work because the cancerous cells are in the way.

There are two types of cancer:

- **Cancer that forms a tumour.** Abnormal masses of cells called tumours are found in building-block cells, like those of the breast, lung, prostate, and skin. These masses of cells kill off surrounding cells as they grow.
- **Cancer that doesn't form a tumour.** Cancer of the blood cells doesn't form a tumour but rather happens when white blood cells—the cells that protect you when you're sick—grow out of control.

Types of tumours

- **Malignant.** The term used to describe tumours that spread because the cells are cancerous.
- **Benign.** The term used to describe tumours that do not spread and are not cancerous.

Types of breast cancer

1. Non-invasive breast cancer

Location: Cells of the breast ducts, called DCIS or ductal carcinoma in situ, meaning "staying in the same place."

Chance of spreading: None.

Risk: If DCIS is not treated it may turn invasive in months or years.

Treatment: Surgery or trials.

2. Invasive breast cancer

A. Invasive ductal (most common)

Location: Cells of the breast ducts.

Chances of spreading: Moderate.

Risk: May develop from other types of breast cancer such as tubular, medullary, papillary, cribriform, and mucinous.

B. Invasive lobular cancer (second-most common)

Location: Cells that line the milk sacs.

Chances of spreading: Classic lobular is slow-spreading; pleomorphic lobular is fast-spreading.

Risk: More common in post-menopausal women.

3. Invasive mixed cancer

A combination of ductal and lobular cancer cells.

4. Inflammatory breast cancer

Location: Lymph vessels in breast.

Chances of spreading: High, and aggressive.

Risk: Very rare.

5. Phyllodes tumour

Location: Connective tissue of the breast.

Chances of spreading: Very rare.

Risk: Most phyllodes tumours are benign and account for less than one percent of breast cancers.

Terms to know

Bone scan. A bone scan is like an X-ray for your bones. When you get a bone scan, technicians inject a very small amount of radioactive tracer into a vein. The tracer gets taken up by the bone and the radiologist can see if there is abnormal activity, which may indicate cancer. Your doctor might order a bone scan before you begin any cancer treatment, to get an idea of the condition of your bones. The bone-scan machine is like a tunnel, and it's noisy. You may get a metallic taste in your mouth from the dye.

CT scan. A computed tomography (CT) scan, often called a CAT scan, uses a series of X-ray images taken at different angles to build a three-dimensional picture of the body. A CT scan can be used to look for cancer, internal bleeding, joint injuries, and many other conditions.

Clinical trials. Clinical trials are research trials that test out new and innovative therapies. These help doctors invent better medicine and treatments. Patients can opt in to a clinical trial but, keep in mind, these are experimental and there is no guarantee of positive results.

PET scan. A positron emission tomography (PET) scan is like an X-ray for your organs and tissues. When you get a PET scan, technicians inject a small amount of radioactive tracer into your body and watch it being taken up by the metabolic activity of different parts of the body. Any abnormal activity seen can help detect conditions such as cancer, heart disease, or dementia. A PET scan may be ordered to look for signs of cancer that were not detected by the MRI or mammogram.

Other terms and procedures will be outlined throughout this book.

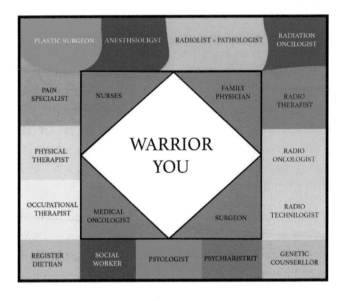

YOUR MEDICAL TEAM:

You. You are at the centre of your team, always remember that. Don't be intimidated. Have the courage to ask questions about your health and your prognosis. Be your own advocate.

Family physician. Your family doctor for your regular or routine medical needs, also called a primary-care physician or general practitioner. This is a physician who practices general medicine. They will take care of common ailments, like a cold or a rash, and they will also coordinate care for your chronic conditions and perform yearly checkups for preventative care.

Medical oncologist. A cancer specialist who helps determine treatment choices like chemotherapy. One or two days, or the same day, before every chemo session, your medical oncologist will see you and discuss how are you coping with drugs and pain.

Surgical Oncologist. A surgeon who specializes in cancer surgeries such as biopsies and tumour removal. Medical, surgical, and radiation oncologists work very closely on your case.

Radiation oncologist. A physician who specializes in radiation therapy. They will determine where the radiation needs to go and the extent of your treatments.

Nurses. There will be team of different designated nurses—from registered nurses to nurse practitioners—with clinical nurse specialties.

Radiologist. A specialist who looks at your imaging, X-rays, ultrasound, and mammogram, and will describe findings in a report to your oncologist.

Pathologist. A specialist who looks at tissues and fluid samples who will write pathology reports about cancer types, grades, and stages.

Plastic surgeon. Also known as a reconstructive surgeon. Body parts affected by cancer, such as breasts, can be operated on to restore them to their original appearance. Reconstruction can happen at the same time of your surgery, or after. You can discuss options with your plastic surgeon.

Anesthesiologist. A specialist who puts you to sleep before your surgery.

Pain specialist. You may ask for a pain specialist if your pain is affecting your ability to maintain your daily activities.

Physical therapist. Teaches you techniques to strengthen your muscles after surgery.

Occupational therapist. Helps you recover ability needed for everyday living.

Registered dietitian. Helps you to introduce and/or maintain a healthy and balanced diet.

Radiation technologist. Is trained for positioning patients for X-rays and mammograms, and takes the pictures that will be sent to your radiologist.

Radiation therapist. A trained technician who works with the radiation oncologist who assists patients to position their bodies during radiation and administers radiation treatments.

Genetic counsellor. Arranges the genetic testing and explains the results.

Social worker. Helps you with emotional, financial, childcare, and family issues, etc. Some social workers who specialize in cancer can even answer your questions, provide counselling, and find you support groups in the community.

Psychologist. Someone you can talk to privately, outside your home and family. They're important, because some days you'll have things to say that you might not want your family to hear.

Psychiatrist. Helps you with mental-health and behavioural disorders and can provide you with prescriptions as well.

- Chapter 3 -
Testing

Mammogram.

A mammogram is an X-ray image of the breast. When you get a mammogram, your breast is placed between two plastic plates that are pressed together to help flatten out the breast tissue. Then the X-ray is taken. This sounds painful, but it's not too bad!

There are two types of mammograms. One is called a screening mammogram. These are usually done for women between 50 and 75, every two years. Both breasts are examined in this type of mammogram. By doing the screening on a regular basis, breast images can be compared for changes over time.

The other type is called a diagnostic mammogram. These are done when there is a concern about the breast tissue: for instance, a lump is found, or there is nipple discharge.

What to expect:

As with an ultrasound, you'll be taken into a change stall and given a gown. When you change into the gown, remember to take off your bra. Again, it's a good idea to wear a two-piece outfit. Also, do not apply deodorant the day of your mammogram. You'll wait in the change stall until you're called by a technician.

For the mammogram, you'll need to stand very close to the machine. (Don't worry, the technician will help you with all the positioning). Your breast will be placed on the bottom plastic plate, which will feel cool or even cold. It will feel like your breast is being handled as though not attached to your body, and there will be a pulling sensation. When the second plate is lowered onto the breast there will be pressure, to flatten the tissue out for a better picture. It will be uncomfortable, but only for about a minute. Just keep reminding yourself that this is an important procedure to find cancer.

They usually take at least two images of each breast, but they can take up to four images at different angles. The most common images are with the breast flattened horizontally and at an angle.

On September 5th, 2017, I went to Credit Valley Hospital for my mammogram. I was stressed, frustrated, and depressed. But somewhere deep inside, I found the strength to be brave and think positive. Maybe the lumps were benign.

They were so good and kind at the clinic. There were women of all ages there, and all of us were wondering where we were going to end up. What disease would they find? How far along would it be?

I was taken to a change stall and given a gown to put on that opened at the front. Then I sat there and waited for my name to be called.

The sonographer was pretty friendly. She gave me instructions, then placed my breast between the two plates of the machine, cranking the plates down so they pressed my breast flat. She took pictures, did some adjustments, and took more pictures.

After, I was taken into a different room for a second ultrasound.

Yes, it was breast cancer. It had gone to my lymph nodes.

A biopsy was booked for the following Wednesday. My son's birthday was that Monday. We had a little party in the park with his friends. All I could think was, Will I live to see his next birthday?

Biopsy.

A biopsy is a procedure in which cells and/or tissues are collected for microscopic examination. Most biopsies are done with a needle (a "needle biopsy") inserted into the breast to pick out a piece of tissue. They may or may not use a local anesthetic—freezing—like the dentist. Some biopsies are surgical biopsies, where a larger piece of tissue is removed.

What to expect:

For either biopsy, you may get an ultrasound, mammogram, or MRI first, so the area where they think the tumour is located can be marked.

For a fine-needle biopsy, the needle is so fine that the doctor may choose not to use local anesthetic, as the freezing needle may prove more painful than the biopsy needle.

For a core-needle biopsy, the doctor will usually use a local anesthetic, for which they will apply a numbing cream before putting the freezing needle in. You'll feel a burning sensation as the anesthetic enters your body, but this will quickly subside as the freezing takes effect and the area goes numb.

Once you're frozen, you'll only feel pressure as the biopsy needle enters your body. This isn't a pleasant feeling. Any woman can remember when the doctor told us we would feel a slight pressure when they did a pap test on our cervix. Not pleasant. But it only takes a couple of minutes and then it's over.

For a surgical biopsy, you'll likely be in an operating room and be given a general anesthetic. This will put you to sleep and you'll wake up after the procedure is over.

After your biopsy, the incision area will be painful once the freezing wears off. Keep the area clean and use ice to help reduce bruising. An icepack covered with a thin cloth fits nicely, tucked inside your bra.

The most painful part about a biopsy is waiting for the results.

The hospital said I would be OK to drive myself home after the biopsy, but I ended up having my cousin drive me. This turned out to be a good thing!

To start, they did an ultrasound on my breast and marked where they determined the lumps were.

Then, they froze the area where the needle would go in. I am not good with needles. I hope others don't struggle with the biopsy procedure as much as I did.

The needle for the freezing hurt like hell, as expected for such a sensitive area. At first, the anesthesiologist gave me just two needles for the freezing, but then she gave me a third needle because I said the area still wasn't numb. She wouldn't give me any more after that.

I screamed when they put the biopsy needle in. It sounded and felt like a staple gun when they grabbed and removed the tissue: tack-tack-tack. You have to stay still and quiet the whole time. It was excruciating.

After the procedure, they checked to make sure they had collected enough tissue to examine. Mine was all good. No second round of torture for me!

I was told to get up and go home, but I felt so dizzy and couldn't get up from the bed. They were rushing me out so the next person could have their procedure. I got up, very unsteady, and tried to walk to the waiting room to meet my cousin, but I was unsuccessful. In the biopsy area, it still felt like there were needles pinching me. The pain was sharp; my head was going round and round. One of the girls helped me to a changeroom and brought my cousin to me.

My cousin was worried, seeing me in such a condition. Her sister had been through the same thing. We sat for a moment. I could see the fear in her eyes. We were both single moms, and she understood the uncertainty I was facing. Finally, she took my right arm and guided me out to the car. We stopped at Tim Hortons and got my favourite, French Vanilla, to get my sugar levels and my spirits up.

I had a follow-up appointment exactly one week later.

Useful tips when going for a biopsy

- Take someone with you to drive you back.
- Don't take aspirin or other blood thinners because that might increase the bruising.
- Empty your bladder before going into the room as it may take a long time for your procedure.
- Bring a light snack or some change so you can buy a snack, as you may need extra energy after the procedure.
- If they use a dye, drink plenty of water afterwards to help clear it from your system.

After the biopsy, I was sent for an MRI to see how much the cancer had spread.

MRI.

Magnetic resonance imagining (MRI) uses magnetic waves and pulses of radiofrequency waves (not the same as radiation) to take three-dimensional pictures of the body. It's very good for taking pictures of soft tissues so it's good for seeing cancer tumours.

What to expect:

Because of the magnetic nature of this machine, you'll need to let your doctor know if you have any metal implants, including a copper IUD or tattoos (some inks contain metal). Of course, you'll also need to remove all jewelry before going into the MRI. As with all these big-machine scans, you'll need to put on a gown.

There might be a dye injection, depending on what the doctors are looking for.

This machine is very loud and can be frightening if you're claustrophobic. Expect to hear a series of loud thumps as the machine goes through its processes.

You'll lie on a table, which will be moved into the machine. Your job will be to stay as still as possible. They might take you out to reposition you during the procedure.

The MRI machine was like a tunnel. I closed my eyes and started chanting my mantra while they were setting me up. Throughout the exam I kept my eyes closed, which kept me from panicking about the fact that I was inside a machine! Halfway through, they pulled me out, injected a dye, and moved me back. Everyone feels different effects from the dye. Some have a metallic taste in their mouth, some smell the dye, and some feel warm waves in the genital area.

Useful tips for an MRI

- Keep your eyes closed during the procedure.
- Take someone with you.
- Don't wear any jewelry.
- Ask for a blanket.
- Tell the technician if you have any metal, such as an implant, in your body.
- Don't wear nylon clothing.

- Chapter 4 -
Be Your Own Advocate

Know your body and listen to it. No one else can advocate for it better than you. Cancer brings a lot of challenges, and making decisions can be confusing. Take the time to be thoughtful and reasonable. Don't make decisions out of fear.

Any cancer patient has the right to choose their own doctor, lawyer, and healthcare team.

Getting the diagnosis

When I walked into that family doctor's clinic in Brampton on August 30th, I was making the decision to finally stand up for myself. Enough was enough. No more Googling my symptoms! I self-advocated and demanded a physical. I guess I was blessed that, at that point, my symptoms were visible on the surface of my body.

When my family doctor suggested I do medical imaging at Brampton Civic Hospital, I didn't want to take a chance. After what I had been through, something told me to choose Credit Valley instead. It was the right decision to get out of Brampton Health Services and try something better.

Finding the right surgeon

On September 20th I had a follow-up appointment with a surgeon at Credit Valley Hospital. He was short, red-faced, and unfit, and reminded me of a butcher more than a surgeon. His biggest concerns seemed to be to get me to sign a consent form, and to get the dates down for my operation. But I was already on the road to self-advocacy. I had a list of questions before I was going to sign anything.

Suffice it to say, some doctors do not like it when patients ask questions. But I refused to sign the consent form.

I wanted more information about my diagnosis and treatment. I didn't trust anyone after what it took for me to get a proper diagnosis. This was my body, and my decision.

I was also in contact with a friend of a friend, an oncologist practising in the U.S., to get a second opinion.

The next week I had a second follow-up with the red-faced surgeon at Credit Valley. This time, my co-worker Poonam came with me for the drive. Poonam's dad had had breast cancer, so she was a good choice to support me for the visit.

I checked in at reception and got my wristband with my date of birth and details. After 10 minutes a nurse came and took us inside. We waited in a small room for the surgeon. It felt like a jail cell.

The surgeon approached and began with the paperwork in his hand. "So, have you decided? Now, let's sign the consent form."

He was pushing me way too hard to sign this document.

"Why are you not signing the consent form?" he asked. "You have a life-threatening disease!"

At this point I felt so threatened and pressured that I began crying. I asked the red-faced surgeon for earlier bone-scan and CT-scan appointments, but he said he didn't have time to "shop around" to find these dates. I was very disappointed.

The Brampton physicians didn't diagnose my cancer at its early stages, and now the red-faced surgeon at Credit Valley was all too eager to chop off my breast! If you're in this situation, don't doubt yourself. Keep away from brutal, rude butchers who just want to cut you up and claim fees from a health-insurance plan.

Poonam suggested I sign the consent form, and if I changed my mind, I could withdraw it. But the red-faced surgeon said I couldn't do that. He said once it was signed, only he could make changes. I felt that, if I signed, there would be no escape from this butcher. I just wanted to get up and leave, but instead I sat there and thought about how to reply without being rude. I finally told him I needed more time to think about it.

He said, "Why do you not understand you have a life-threatening disease?"

This was the second time in less than ten minutes I was reminded that I had a life-threatening disease. It was not easy to digest. I started to think about how critical my cancer was and that I was going to die. But I had to stop my mind from wandering.

We left the hospital, quite upset at the surgeon's harsh words. I don't know what karma or misdeed was haunting me at the time, but I decided that this surgeon would not be my surgeon. When I look back today, it's clear that quitting that surgeon and facility was my best act of self-advocacy.

Later that day, the red-faced surgeon's office called me with appointments on October 16th and 17th for my body and CT scan. Those dates felt too far off; I was worried the cancer would spread. And I was right. Within these three months, my cancer had moved to its second stage due to the negligence of my family physicians.

I stuck to my gut feelings. I'd been scouring YouTube looking for all kinds of information. There was a lot of stuff about naturopathy, from bitter almonds to wheatgrass, carrot juice to B17. The list was never-ending.

I ended up calling clinics in Mexico to find out what they could do and how they would do it. I wanted to know the survival rate of their treatment, as it would cost $70,000 to $90,000. I then sought the advice of the oncologist I'd been consulting in the U.S. He was truthful and helped me decide on conventional medical treatment. My emotions were extremely up and down, like the giant rollercoaster at Canada's Wonderland.

I decided to go to Princess Margaret Cancer Centre in Toronto to see what they could do for me. I had hope leading up to that visit.

My general practitioner's office couldn't do much but say they'd call me back once they received my reports from Princess Margaret. I ended up calling Princess Margaret and found out they had only received a referral from a doctor at a walk-in clinic, one who hadn't seen me in June.

I Googled Princess Margaret Cancer Centre in Toronto for breast cancer. Dr. McCready's name came up at the top of the search:

Dr. McCready holds the Gattuso Chair in Breast Surgical Oncology at Princess Margaret Hospital and is Head of the Breast Cancer Centre at Princess Margaret Cancer Centre. He is principal investigator of the National Surgical Adjuvant Breast and Bowel Project at the Princess Margaret Hospital site and is a member of the Breast Site Executive of the National Institute of Canada Clinical Trials Group.

Somehow I found a number to call. Luckily, my call was answered, and I got hold of Dr. McCready's assistant. I'll call her Alice. She was my angel and still is.

Alice booked my initial appointment in September, but because they didn't get any images, they didn't follow up. I had to go to Credit Valley myself to collect them, and then emailed them to Princess Margaret, so my new medical team could look at my case prior to my visit.

On September 29th I drove to the hospital, and Dee, a friend and wife of a cancer survivor, met me there. We checked in at reception where a pretty voice called, "Jag!"

I wondered who knew my nickname at the hospital. It was Alice! She gave me a big hug. What a warm first connection with this new hospital.

Alice took Dee and me to a room. She explained that Dr. McCready was away but that we would meet with another surgeon. I was instructed to change into a gown and wait for the surgeon to arrive.

When the surgeon came, Dee asked her a couple of questions on my behalf. The surgeon did a physical exam and told me about next steps. As Dr. Gupta from the U.S. had explained, this surgeon was going to pursue a neo-adjuvant treatment to stop the spread of the cancer before surgery. Neo-adjuvant treatment means treatment before surgery.

This new surgeon was a star. She didn't ask or force me to sign a consent form, unlike the Credit Valley surgeon. Her manner helped me to trust her, the treatment, and the hospital. I felt I was in safe, honest hands.

Self-advocacy had got me into a hospital considered one of the top-five cancer-research hospitals in the world.

Breast reconstruction

My next self-advocacy move concerned breast reconstruction.

My reconstruction surgery consultation was held at the Women's College Hospital in Toronto.

The surgeon was so down-to-earth. He listed all the options. He even said, "Even though reconstruction is covered by Ontario Health Insurance Plan, it is completely your choice if you want it now, later, or never."

I respect this surgeon so much, but I chose to live with one breast and one prosthesis. I was just so nervous about surgery in any form. I had never had surgery before. Going to sleep with an anesthetic was too scary. The thought of never waking up terrified me.

Extended hospital stay

My final self-advocacy move was to ask if they would let me stay in the hospital for a night post-surgery. I was scared to go home. What if something went wrong? They agreed to this request, which left me feeling comfortable and relieved.

Turn your words into wisdom.
- **Oprah Winfrey**

- Chapter 5 -
Understanding Your Reports

Many people don't take the time to understand their full diagnosis and, instead, let their illness lay shrouded in mystery.

Take the time to read your reports. Ask questions. Once you know what is happening in your body, you'll understand your treatment, too.

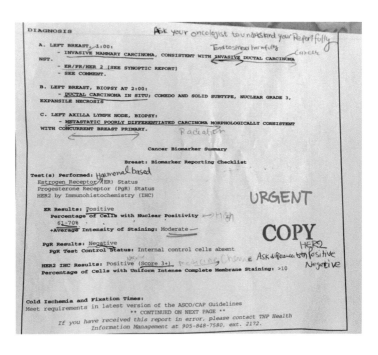

Here is a list of some of the items you might see in your report.

Hormone receptors for breast cancer

There are two types of hormone receptors they measure when diagnosing breast cancer.

1. Estrogen receptor (ER)

2. Progesterone receptor (PgR)

If one or both of these receptors are present in breast tissue, the cancer is considered hormone-receptor positive.

Roughly two out of three breast cancers are hormone-receptor positive. This type of cancer grows slowly and responds to hormonal therapy.

Invasive mammary carcinoma

This is when the cancer (carcinoma) has passed through the cells of the milk ducts or lobules and has invaded other tissues.

HER2

HER2 stands for human epidermal growth factor receptor 2, a growth-promoting protein. A tumour with a high level of protein is called a HER2 positive tumour. You can see this in my report (above). This type of tumour tends to grow rapidly. A drug that targets the HER2 protein may be used in your treatment.

Cancer grades vs. cancer stages

Cancer grades.	Cancer stages.
Describe how the cancer cells look and how different they are from normal cells. Establishing the grade of cancer cells helps doctors predict how fast they will grow.	Describe how far the cancer has spread, both from the perspective of tumour size and from its point of origin.
Grade 1: Low grade. Cells are healthy and normal and grow slow.	**T:** Breast tumour. T0, TIS, T1, T2, T3, T4
Grade 2: Intermediate grade.	**N:** Cancer has spread to lymph nodes. N0, N1, N2, N3
Grade 3: Serious and rapid growth.	**M:** Cancer has spread to other parts of the body, for instance, the lungs or the brain. M1, M1

Blood tests

Blood tests are done to find out many things about you, including your general state of health. Blood tests can measure how well your different organs are performing, and how your treatment is progressing. A blood test can identify some diseases and show if you have an infection.

Here are some common types of blood tests.

Complete blood count

This test looks at all the cells in your blood.

- Red blood cells carry oxygen and nutrients to your cells. Hemoglobin (Hgb) in your red blood cells carries oxygen. Lack of Hgb makes you feel tired and short of breath.

- White blood cells (WBCs) are the cells of your immune system. They fight infection. If your WBC count is too low or too high, you might be at risk for infections. If your WBC count is down, you might be given antibiotics to help prevent and fight off infection.

- Neutrophils are a special type of white blood cell. They are the first cells to fight infection. As with white blood cells, if your neutrophils are found to be too low, you may be at risk for infections, and your doctor may prescribe antibiotics.

- Platelets are blood cells that form a block when you're bleeding from a cut or bruise. A low platelet count increases the risk of bleeding. Signs of low platelet count include easy bruising, lots of bruising, bleeding that does not stop (like a nose bleed), and blood in the urine. Sometimes a blood transfusion may be needed to help with a low platelet count.

Electrolytes

This test will measure the levels of important minerals in your body. Electrolytes control many functions, including nerve reactions and muscle movements. They exist in all the fluids in your body. The most common electrolytes are sodium (Na), potassium (K), calcium (Ca), and magnesium (Mg).

Creatinine

This test will measure the amount of creatinine in your blood as a way of checking your kidney function. Creatinine is what is left over when your body makes energy from food. Your kidneys remove creatinine from the blood. If the creatinine levels in your blood are high, it may mean your kidneys aren't functioning properly.

- Chapter 6 -
Dos and Don'ts

Here are some dos and don'ts to keep in mind as you self-advocate through your cancer journey.

Patients

Get a second opinion. Your first experience as a cancer patient might not be good. If you're not comfortable with your doctor or your diagnosis, get a second opinion. Peace of mind is a must during this whole process. You do not want any diagnostic mistakes. Personally, I'm glad that I did my research and contacted Dr. Gupta for a second opinion. After all, the red-faced surgeon didn't even mention neo-adjuvant chemotherapy. Thank God my second surgeon did.

Ask questions and understand your diagnosis. Double-check the information you're given. It's OK to ask questions. Read your reports and learn about what is happening to you.

Allow yourself to have feelings. It's OK to be sad, depressed, and anxious. Humans are full of emotions. If you're sick like this, you're going to be hit with some intense feelings. Don't worry; they're natural. Don't suppress them. Cry when you want. Yell when you need to.

You might be wondering why someone who says she courageously beat cancer is telling you to cry. Well, we women feel a lot lighter after a good cry! We have to experience our emotions to get over them. And our emotions are powerful. Feel that power inside you and let it out.

Fight with style. Even hair loss can be stylish. You'll have smooth legs and underarms. Imagine: a Brazilian without the pain! I thought I looked sexier and more beautiful than ever when I was bald. This kind of positive attitude made me feel happy and gave me the courage to keep fighting.

At the time, I was volunteering at the Chinguacousy Wellness Centre in Brampton. I asked if I could wear one of their wigs. It was a challenge to find one that matched my natural hair colour because most of them were blond, but eventually I was successful. When I wore it, everyone thought I had a new hairstyle. I was in the early stages of chemo, but nobody knew. People loved it! The compliments just kept coming. The wig also helped keep my head warm during the winter months.

After chemo, my hair started to grow back. I had my surgery in March. In April and May I looked so young, with my spiky hair growing out, so I stopped wearing wigs and scarves. I just went around bald. I got some nasty looks from people in my community, especially when my two boys walked with me wearing their turbans. But who cares about hair? I wasn't depressed anymore. Instead, I got a kick out of being brave and bald. I felt stylish, and that gave me courage.

Be patient. The one thing cancer taught me was patience. Slow down and enjoy what you have in life. This is easier said than done, but believe me, it's a valuable tool. The calmer you are during and after your treatment, the quicker you'll recover. As long as you understand the basics of your diagnosis and treatment, you can move forward, step-by-step, with patience and control.

Appoint your caregivers. In most cases, your caregiver will be your partner or your spouse. If not, maybe a close friend, a parent, sibling, or one of your children. I suggest you build your care team as soon as possible. Remember that your income may be limited, so visitors from overseas might not be a feasible option.

You need people you can really rely on. When people are emotional, they make big promises they can't practically commit to. You must be clear when you're recruiting help that you may look good before you start treatment, but you'll get sick, and need your caregivers to step up. You need to make sure those people know you're counting on them.

Talk to other cancer patients. Try not to feel alone. Cancer happens to a lot of people. There are a lot of experienced warriors out there. You'll make new friends at hospitals, too. Some volunteers are survivors, and they have stories to tell.

Know your fertility. Fertility wasn't especially important in my case because I already had kids, but if you don't and you think you may want children later on, you must ask your oncologist before starting any treatment. You may be able to preserve your eggs so there's the possibility of having kids.

Eat in small portions. Eating wisely helped me during chemotherapy. I had breakfast before 7 AM so my stomach was empty before my chemo infusion. I highly recommend this. Also, bring water with you. You can have crackers and water during your treatment, but don't eat heavy Indian foods with lots of meat. Don't eat spicy foods or raw meat either. I recommend boiled or steamed vegetables with rice for the first couple of days after a chemo treatment. You might also find interim fasting helps settle your digestive system.

Another good way to keep your stomach calm and your body strong is to drink a lot of fluids. Try freshly squeezed juices, like carrot juice, coconut juice, or wheatgrass.

Make sure to avoid sugary products. If you want something sweet, try natural honey.

Take control of what you can and forget about the rest. Not all things will be in your control, so don't worry about them. Once I knew my diagnosis and treatment plan, I stopped worrying. I focused on productive things and refused to waste energy on what I couldn't control.

Guru Nanak Ji says, "God is there to worry about us; he even created the sea life and provided them with food." These lines help me find the strength not to worry.

Caregivers

Listen to your patient with your mouth shut. Whether you're a partner, sibling, or child, you must shut your big or small mouth and listen to the patient. I took someone to the lawyer with me to help me with my will. When we were done, I wanted to have something to eat. The person laughed at me and said, "Why are you worrying about eating? Sooner or later, cancer is death."

Don't say you know how they feel. You're not a patient; you don't know their pain. Don't say you know how they feel unless you've been through it yourself.

Be positive. My surgeon said, "The doctor can only do so much. The rest is up to the patients, including how positive and happy they are. The more positive you are, the better your immune system fights the disease. Your treatment works better." Your positive attitude around the patient can help them heal.

Don't ask if they need help; just do it. Be there to help the person. They have limited energy to help themselves and don't always know how to ask for what they need. Be proactive. You could buy groceries, make dinner, take care of their kids, do household chores, drive them to appointments, or simply offer moral support.

Be considerate about what you say. Sometimes people tell stories without thinking of the other person's feelings and based on unknown sources or hearsay. Don't gossip either!

Because I had lost my husband, most people who called or visited talked about my loss instead of my cancer. This was uncomfortable for me; it felt like they thought I was going to die, too.

Help them laugh. I found laughter was a natural healer. If you're a caregiver, talk to the person about their childhood memories, or whatever else might make them smile. My sister made me laugh by telling stories about our funny uncle and the silly things we'd done together, like how she used to cheat on her exams.

Get them out of the house. It helped me so much when my friends and work colleagues took me out for dinner or coffee. It distracted me from aches, pains, and depression.

Don't share your personal stress. If you're unsettled emotionally, financially, or in any other way, don't put your burden on the cancer patient's shoulder. They need you, not your stress.

- Chapter 7 -
Neoadjuvant Therapy

Neoadjuvant therapy is the coordinated treatment plan you go through before you have surgery. "Adjuvant" means "in addition to." In the case of cancer treatment, it refers to what happens in addition to surgery. It's sometimes referred to as pre-operative therapy and is usually for patients with high-risk, locally advanced breast cancer. The goal is to shrink the tumour(s) before surgery. Neoadjuvant therapy can include hormone therapy, chemotherapy, and radiation.

My neoadjuvant therapy consisted of chemotherapy. I had six chemotherapy sessions before my mastectomy, starting in October. My treatment drugs were FEC-Docetaxel, Anthracycline, and Trastuzumab (Herceptin).

Chemotherapy

Chemotherapy.

Chemotherapy is when drugs are used to kill cancer cells. The drugs work by attacking rapidly growing cells, so, while they kill cancer cells, they can also kill the cells that make hair and line the digestive system. This is why chemotherapy can cause patients to get sick to their stomachs or lose their hair.

Chemotherapy is used in two situations: to treat active cancer or to reduce the recurrence of cancer in people who are believed to be disease-free. In breast cancer, the majority of people who receive treatment receive it preventatively.

Neoadjuvant chemotherapy is for specific, faster growing cancers, especially those that are hormone and HER2 positive.

Doctors prescribe different chemotherapy drugs depending on the kind of tumour you have. The treatments also vary in intensity, with patients infused weekly, biweekly, or every three weeks. The most standard way of delivering chemotherapy is to give larger doses every two or three weeks. The choice is based on logistical differences, the number of visits required, the side effects the patient is experiencing, the age of the patient, and whether the patient has any other medical problems. There are no one-size-fits-all chemo plans.

Chemotherapy drugs are often administered intravenously through a port, catheter, or PICC line. But some chemotherapies are in pill form. Most breast cancer treatments are intravenous.

Chemotherapy before surgery can be very effective. It can reduce the size of the tumours and reduce spread. FEC-Docetaxel is commonly used in the treatment of breast cancer.

FEC-Docetaxel is a name for a bunch of drugs combined into a cocktail: 5-fluorouracil, epirubicin, and cyclophosphamide, plus Docetaxel. These drugs target and kill cells that are rapidly dividing. Usually, you get three treatments of the FEC and then three treatments of just the Docetaxel.

Anthracycline is an antibiotic used in chemotherapy that stops a cell from making copies of its DNA, which means it can't divide into new cells.

The side effects of chemotherapy are different for every drug. Some cause lowered white blood cell count, increasing the risk for infection. Others cause nausea. Others cause reactions at the infusion site. Depending on the type of chemotherapy, different drugs may be included in the treatment in addition to the chemotherapy to help treat these side effects. For instance, some chemotherapies cause nausea and require medication to treat it; others may require a steroid to help treat reactions they cause.

Targeted therapy

Anything that is used that has a specific marker on the cancer is considered targeted therapy.

Trastuzumab (Herceptin) is a type of targeted therapy that targets HER2. Hormone therapy is also a type of targeted therapy because it targets estrogen. Targeted therapies are less toxic than chemotherapy because they are so targeted. Herceptin has few side effects but can cause some heart-function issues.

Some chemotherapies can be combined with targeted therapies. If the chemo has similar side effects to the targeted therapy, they are generally not given at the same time. Because of Herceptin's heart-function issues, it's generally not combined with Anthracyclines, which are also associated with heart problems.

What to expect

Because chemotherapy is repeated several times, you'll most likely have some kind of semi-permanent port installed in your body. If your cancer is only in one breast, the port will be installed on the opposite side.

The first chemo session is often the least eventful. Make sure you take all the medications that you're prescribed. The anti-nauseants and painkillers make a huge difference in how you feel after your treatment. Symptoms can become worse in subsequent treatments, as the chemo drugs build up in your system. This is where you might experience digestive issues, hair loss, changes in your nails and skin, fatigue, and even mouth sores. Also, your periods might stop.

Some people say the worst part about chemotherapy is the brain fog or "chemo brain." Memory loss, struggling to find words, or trouble staying organized or learning new things are some of the ways chemotherapy seems to affect the brain. This fog can last well after your treatments are completed.

As the start of my chemo neared, Nev, my cousin from Indianapolis, arrived with her husband and their two sweet daughters. I could clearly see the fear in their faces. I advised them to get refreshed so we could go visit the CN Tower and Nathan Phillips Square, because, after my chemo, I may not be up for much. We also drove past the hospital so they could get familiar with parking and such. It was a lovely day. In my mind, I was wondering if I would ever see my nieces again. I wanted to make their trip memorable.

First chemo session – October 16th, 2017

- FEC
- Fatigue and mild nausea in first few days
- Constipation followed by loose stools
- Some bone pain that subsided spontaneously
- Naproxen prescribed for pain.

October 17th, a Thursday, was my first chemo day. Before leaving, I said my routine prayer and asked God to help me stay strong and healthy. We left home early to avoid traffic on the way to Toronto.

At Princess Margaret Cancer Centre, the volunteers were so welcoming and really put me at ease. Walking through those doors, I was filled with positivity. My energy was good. I looked forward to the initial consultation with my oncologist and surgeon. I sat in the waiting room for only about 10 minutes before I was called to register. I was then issued a wristband, with my name, birthdate, and Medical Record Number (MRN).

I waited about an hour to start my treatment. I sat in a recliner and wore a loose top with an opening at the front that made it much easier for the nurses to run the catheter into the right side of my breast. The nurse cleaned the area and then poked in my port. I screamed in pain and broke into tears. Seeing me like this, Nev got teary, too. She had to leave for a few seconds. That made me even more emotional.

It's amazing how emotionally connected Nev and I were, even though we hadn't seen each other in ten years. Whatever fears and misunderstandings we had dissolved. Love was everywhere. At least cancer was bringing us together. I forgot the pain soon enough.

The nurse flushed the port before administering the chemo and told me that I would get hot flashes. I was given some ice to suck on to keep me cool and to help prevent ulcers. I also put my toes and fingers in ice.

This first session took about an hour and a half. It went well, and I could walk afterwards. I didn't fall or need to go to bed. It did slow me down though, so I went home and rested. I skipped my lunch and had boiled rice, potatoes, and peas for dinner.

The following day, I had to go back to the hospital for a checkup and to get an injection of Grastofill, an immune-system booster. I would have one injection at the hospital and the remaining six would be administered later at home.

After the treatment at the hospital, we made a trip to Centre Island. That was a happy time. For just a few moments, I forgot about my cancer and the effects of chemo.

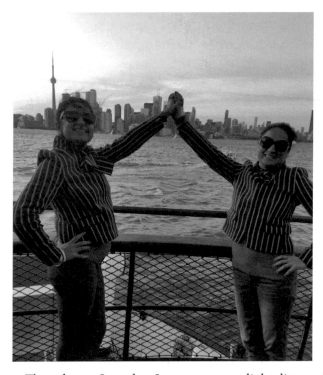

From Thursday to Saturday, I was on a very light diet, and I drank a lot of liquids so that my digestive system could adjust to the chemo medicines. I also fasted intermittently: this is supposed to help with immunity and digestion.

My faith in love and God got stronger every day. I would start my days with a shower and prayers. I tried to stay independent and make my own breakfasts, and I kept cooking for my kids. At first, it seemed like chemo would be manageable. My mission to live life to the best was still on.

My area MP, Ruby Sahota, knew what I was going through. I had expressed my wish to visit Ottawa, and she was generous enough to offer me a visit to Parliament. We drove to Ottawa in the evening and got there around midnight. During this time, I was shedding hair like a shaggy dog. It was falling out and sticking to the car seats, headrest, and pillows—pretty much everywhere—which meant I had to wear a headscarf for the visit.

We stayed at a hotel. The next morning, we got formally dressed. My hair was like a bird's nest. I couldn't comb it because it stuck together. My head started to ache, and my eyes started to strain. We went through security, and Ruby met us in the corridor. We waited for Minister of Defence, Harjit Singh Sajjan.

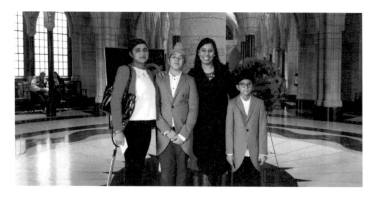

Once we came back from Ottawa, I decided to get my head shaved. It was autumn and, while the leaves weren't falling yet, my hair sure was.

I sat in a barber's chair. My friend talked with the barber to make sure that all the tools he used were sanitized. As soon as I sat in the chair with my head down, tears started to flow. When the barber asked why I was crying, my friend told him I was going through cancer, and then the barber started crying himself. He didn't even charge me for his services.

Hair loss can be very upsetting for a woman. Mine fell out after my first chemo session. I recommend that you get your head shaved before your hair starts falling out!

Second chemo session – November 9th, 2017

- FEC
- Pain controlled by Naproxen
- ECG (heart monitor) showed normal results
- Nausea controlled by Pantoprazole
- Hair loss

I decided to go bald to my next chemo session. At the hospital, we all felt like one community. We were very much connected. There were no stares or dirty looks. Just love and sympathy.

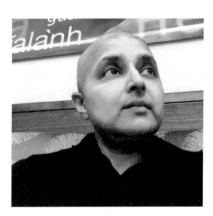

But people without cancer would stare and give me dirty looks. Once, I was confronted at Shoppers Drug Mart with my sons, who have head buns. A Punjabi guy asked me if the boys were mine. He asked if I was Punjabi and wondered why I was bald. I told him I was currently undergoing treatment, not trying to be a fashion icon. He was Sikh, too, but he was clean-shaven and had his hair cut. Who was he to bug me about looking Sikh? Unfortunately, there are always narrow-minded people who will judge you.

I had fun at the Armani Store in the Eaton Centre. I tried on different shapes and shades of sunglasses. I loved the feeling of modelling at such a fancy store. There I was, a girl who was fighting cancer, intoxicated with chemo drugs. Seeing myself as an Armani model was a great triumph.

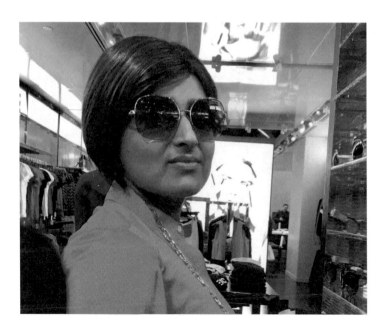

> **Third chemo session – November 30th, 2017**
>
> - FEC
> - Tumours responding well. Large mass now less than 1 cm
> - Normal appetite and sleeping well

For my third treatment, my middle biological sister from New Zealand came to support me. I was so alone for so long that seeing my sister boosted my energy, because she felt I had been a great role model, mentor, and supporter for her. Her presence gave me more courage, which gave me the strength to overcome the side effects of chemo. The happiness of living life in the moment cannot be described, only experienced.

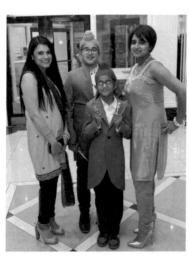

I didn't have anyone to drive me to the hospital, so I drove my sister and me. That same evening, I drove back and went to a Christmas party at Re-Max, my employer, an event I didn't want to miss. I got to wear my favourite dress, necklace, and, of course, my wig. I enjoyed my time with my sister, my kids, and my colleagues. They were all so excited to see me there. They admired my courage in attending. I was full of chemo drugs, but still in my heels, and I didn't trip or fall. The aroma of Indian food was hard to resist, but I controlled myself and didn't eat a bite.

Fourth chemo session – December 21st, 2017

- Docetaxel and Trastuzumab (Herceptin)
- ECG and bloodwork OK
- Experiencing pain. Doctor offered Percocet prescription to help with pain.

My other sister, Raj, her husband, and her son arrived from India. She took good care of me on a daily basis. At this point in the treatment, I was really starting to get worn out. The pain in my bones and joints was unbearable. Raj would make me fresh carrot juice in the morning and sit with me. Her son would come and hug me every day. He was a good distraction in the house. If Raj hadn't come, the last three chemotherapies would have been too hard to cope with. Raj stayed with me until June, when I was almost finished my radiation therapy. Then, they had to move out to Newfoundland to complete their immigration process for permanent residency.

Fifth chemo session – January 11th, 2018

- Docetaxel and Trastuzumab
- ECG and bloodwork OK
- Fatigue when exercising

During this time, I went to the local cancer-wellness centre for yoga and relaxation classes.

I also saw a grief counsellor to deal with my unresolved issues about my husband's death.

I would fall asleep during counselling sessions, yoga, or simply in the middle of the day, as my nights were sleepless. But my sister staying with me helped a lot, physically, emotionally, and morally. I was so eager to get my last chemo session over with and be done with the pain.

> **Sixth and final chemo session – February 1st, 2018**
>
> - Docetaxel and Trastuzumab
> - MRI confirmed cancer's response to treatment, but surgery still required
> - Abnormal lymph node normalized

I am so fortunate to be able to say my neoadjuvant chemotherapy was very successful, and my tumour mass was reduced from 1.7 cm to less than 1 cm in diameter by the time I had completed my third chemo session. I was ready for the next step: surgery.

- Chapter 8 -
Surgery

March 1st, 2018, was my surgery day. I recommend you attend pre-surgery classes if your hospital offers them. It will help you understand the process.

Lumpectomy.

A lumpectomy is surgery to remove a lump in the breast. The surgeon will remove the tumour and some of the healthy surrounding tissue to make sure they get all the cancer. A lumpectomy is also called a segmental excision, a wedge resection, a wide excision biopsy, or a partial mastectomy.

Mastectomy

Simple or total mastectomy

With a simple mastectomy, also called a total mastectomy, the surgeon removes the entire breast: tissue, nipple, areola, and skin.

Modified radical mastectomy

With a modified radical mastectomy, the surgeon removes the entire breast—the same as a simple mastectomy plus underarm lymph nodes and the lining over the muscle tissue beneath the breast.

Who usually gets a modified radical mastectomy? Most people with invasive breast cancer who decide to have mastectomies will receive modified radical mastectomies. This allows for the lymph nodes to be examined to see if the cancer has spread beyond the breast.

Useful tips for going to hospital

Bring/wear:

- Your health insurance card
- Any medication you're on
- Change for drinks and snacks
- A book or magazine
- Sports bra without underwire
- A shawl to cover your top parts
- Slippers or comfortable slip-on shoes (no high heels, laces, or boots)
- Loose clothing that opens in the front

Don't bring/wear:

- Expensive jewelry or watches
- Perfumes, deodorant, or scented lotions

A day prior to your surgery, you'll receive a dye injection to identify the nodes.

Notes

Two intradermal (into the skin) injections using 100 MBq Tc 99-m sulfur colloid particles in the left breast. Lymphatic drainage is visualized in the left axilla with one node identified and marked on the skin for the scheduled resection.

Surgery day – step by step

Vital signs assessment

The first step for booking your surgery is a vital-signs assessment.

Temperature:	37.1 (98.8 F)	
Temperature Route:	oral	
Pulse:	Value:	92
	Unit:	bpm
Pulse Description:	regular	
Resp Rate:	Value:	18
	Unit:	breaths/min
Oxygen (O2) Saturation:	Value:	100
	Unit:	%
Oxygen (O2)/Resp Delivery System:	Room air	
Blood Pressure:	116/82	
Blood Pressure Position:	sitting	

Breast biopsy specimen

After your assessment, they'll do a biopsy using breast-lumpectomy specimen radiography.

Notes

The left axillary specimen demonstrates one complete hook wire in situ with the associated targeted, clipped, malignant level I axillary lymph node for excision.

Results will be verbally phoned to the operating room. Correlation with final surgical pathology is recommended.

Before I started chemo, I had a clip wire (also called a clip marker) inserted to mark the location of my tumour. This helps monitor the size of the tumour to see if it shrinks during chemotherapy.

Mammogram and breast ultrasound

Notes

INDICATION: Planned left mastectomy today. Previously clipped cytology proven malignant level I left axillary lymph node. Present for pre-operative wire localization of previous clip.

PROCEDURE: Informed consent was obtained after discussion emphasizing small risks of bleeding and infection.

I was prepped, draped, and positioned using a sterile technique. Local anesthetic was administered.

Because there were no immediate complications, I was discharged from this department to the care of the operating room.

Surgery

Once you're taken into the operating theatre, you'll be asked for personal information to confirm you are the right patient. Then they will tell you to count numbers after administering the anesthetic. You'll fall asleep during counting and wake up in the recovery room.

Mastectomy surgery takes two to three hours. If you're having breast reconstruction at the same time, it will take longer.

When you wake up you may have a bandage over your breast area and one or more tubes coming out near the surgical site. These tubes drain excess blood and fluid to help in the healing process. They will stay in your body for a week or two. Rather than pain, you'll feel tightness and pinching in the areas where the tissue was removed. You'll also feel the stitches, of course.

I woke up asking for water because my throat was so dry. It took me a couple of hours to regain consciousness. It was scarier for my family than for me.

After surgery, I felt so light, like a burden had been lifted off my shoulder.

Discharge plan

You'll be discharged from the hospital with instructions. If you requested home care, this should start as soon as you get home.

Follow-up instructions for patient should include:

- When to call your family physician or primary-care provider.

- A follow-up appointment date in two to three weeks with your surgeon.

- Instructions for care and cleaning of drain over the next few days or weeks, including how to bathe and shower.

- How to monitor the fluid discharged from the site.

- How to recognize if there is infection at the site.

- Medications you should be taking.

- What foods to eat and what foods to avoid.

- Activities to avoid and exercises that can help you heal.

- When you can resume work, depending on what you do for work.

- Chapter 9 -
Radiation and Hormone Therapy

Radiation Therapy.

Radiation therapy

This type of cancer treatment uses high doses of radiation to safely target and kill cancer cells, effectively shrinking any tumours in your body. Radiation is most often done after surgery or chemotherapy and focuses on the area where there is potential for recurrence.

The radiation used in such therapy is a much higher dose than in X-rays.

What to expect

Your radio-oncologist will tell you how many radiation sittings you'll need.

Before your actual radiation treatment, you'll attend a pre-radiation appointment where technicians will teach you how to breathe and hold your breath for a few seconds at a time. You'll get a chance to practice this breathing technique at this appointment.

The technicians will also do some measurements and mark your body. These marks will help the technicians to set the machine and identify where to focus the radiation beam. There is a risk of damaging some healthy cells during this process.

On treatment day, you'll receive a gown to change into and wait in the change stall until the technician calls your name. Then, you'll follow the technician into a room, where you'll lie down on a table, and your name and date of birth are confirmed.

At this moment, you can ask for a warm blanket.

After setting the machine, the technicians will leave the room. You'll still be able to hear them giving you instructions about when to hold your breath. After the first round, the technicians will come back into the room and reposition the machine, if your radiation involves more than one area.

It doesn't hurt during the process, but your skin will get very sensitive and start to peel and blister afterwards. You have to look after your skin: don't use perfumes or scented lotions. You'll receive instructions or a handout on skincare.

Useful tips for radiation

- Keep the radiated area as clean as possible.
- Don't rub your skin even though it may be itchy.
- Drink as much fluid as you can.
- Don't put any oil or lotions on before going for your radiation treatment.
- Wear loose and comfortable T-shirts.
- I used clarified butter (desi ghee) after treatment to soothe my skin, but don't use it before treatment.

It was a baking hot summer in Toronto. I had 21 sessions of radiation. Having this treatment gave me hot dry skin, other symptoms included burning sensations and peeling.

Hormone Therapy.

Also called hormonal therapy or hormone manipulation, this is a treatment that works with the hormones of the body or artificial hormones to stop cancer-cell growth. Some hormone-therapy drugs will suppress the activity of hormones produced by the cancer cells; some drugs will suppress the actual production of hormones by the cancer cells.

Hormone therapy is used after chemotherapy, after surgery, and often after radiation therapy as well. For cancers that are sensitive to estrogen (hormone positive cancers), which are most breast cancers, hormone therapy can block the estrogen, which can further lower the recurrence of the cancer.

What to expect

Treatments early on can consist of fluid injections, which will likely be combined in your chemo cocktail. Afterwards you'll be given the hormone in pill form.

- Chapter 10 -
Side Effects Of Treatment

No matter what your treatment, chances are you will experience side effects. I certainly did. Be prepared. Here are some of the more common ones.

Hot flashes. All of a sudden, your body starts to produce too much heat. You'll feel your head boiling and your feet on fire. Even in winter, you'll tear off your hat, socks, blankets, jacket—whatever is on your body—just to cool off. Hot flashes are unpredictable. They can happen when you're watching TV, in the middle of the night when you're sleeping, or when you're shopping in the mall.

If you're wearing a wig as I was you'll feel the sweat dripping underneath it. It's such a gross feeling. Once the hot flash has passed, you'll be freezing again.

Part of the reason for your hot flashes might be because your treatment has caused you to go into early menopause, and your hormone levels are messed up. See below.

Infections. Since your white blood cell count can go down because of cancer, or because of chemo, you're more at risk for infection. The earliest warning of an infection is a fever of over 38°C. A digital thermometer is worth buying so you can monitor yourself.

To avoid infection, your caretaker can help you keep your home's hygienic standards above normal. You should also change your bed sheets regularly, use the same washroom (unshared, if possible), use anti-bacterial gel, and stay away from people who are sick or might be carrying germs or viruses.

Anemia. People who are lacking in red blood cells have anemia because their iron is low. The condition makes you tired, weak, and pale. It helps to eat foods high in iron, like green and leafy vegetables, sweet potatoes, prunes, raisins, dried apricots, dried peaches, and beans.

Fatigue. You'll suffer from lack of energy and fatigue for a while, even after you're done your treatment. It helps to eat healthy foods high in protein, iron, and vitamins. Take naps throughout the day, but keep a schedule. Don't be in bed all day, as you won't get any sleep at night. Go sit in the family room and keep yourself distracted. Listen to soothing music. The calmer you stay, the quicker you recover.

Nausea. One of the most common side-effects of chemotherapy is nausea. It helps to eat and drink in small quantities. Guava helped my nausea a lot.

Skin rashes and dryness. Skin rashes and dryness can also be a problem. Your skin gets really dry and can crack. I used clarified butter (desi ghee) after treatment to soothe my skin. Use natural but less fragranted products.

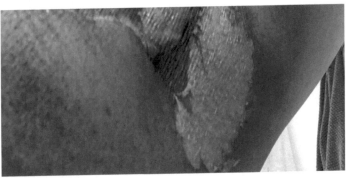

Mouth sores. Chemo can damage the lining of the throat and mouth, causing bleeding and ulcers. Brush after every meal, if possible. You can make your own mouthwash by mixing one cup of warm water with half a teaspoon of salt or baking soda. Swish the mix in your mouth for at least 30 seconds and then spit it out. Don't use commercial mouthwashes because they are strong and harmful during chemo. Your healthcare team will give you some advice as well.

Menopause. Even though menopause tends to happen in your 50s, chemotherapy can bring it on, too. I stopped menstruating after four cycles of chemo. Chemo can also cause vaginal dryness, itchiness, and discomfort—all signs of early menopause.

Brain fog. The most common and long-lasting side effect of treatment is brain fog. Your mind falls asleep in the middle of a conversation. You forget words while talking. It slows you down in many ways. One time, I was so foggy I forgot to take my injections with me after chemotherapy: $1200 worth of medication left behind! I didn't realize it until a nurse called me the next day and told me they were still at the clinic.

Weight changes. When your metabolism slows down after menopause, it's very common to gain weight.

Mood swings. Having low levels of estrogen makes you moody and irritable. People around me found me very unpredictable. I ended up getting panic attacks and anxiety in stressful situations.

Aches and pains. One of the most common side effects is pain in your joints, bones and body. Try natural remedies. Do light yoga. Sit in water. Try meditating, keep yourself calm.

Loss of appetite. You might lose your appetite during chemotherapy. Try light snacks to keep up your energy level. Drink plenty of fluid to keep hydrated. Eat in small portions.

Lack of interest in sex. After menopause, you might feel less interested in sex due to vaginal dryness, hot flashes, fatigue, weakness, and aches. Losing your one breast may make you feel less feminine and embrassed in bed.

- Chapter 11 -
Support Outside The Home

Your cancer journey is your own and part of self-advocacy is taking the initiative to care for yourself. Not everyone at home will be able to give you the support you need when you need it. Don't hesitate to reach out to other resources, there are so many out there.

Wellness centres. Canada has in-house cancer-wellness centres at many of its hospitals. Here, you can find various classes, from healthy-cooking workshops to yoga and meditation.

Look good feel better. This is a two-hour class where you'll learn how to use hygienic make-up application to keep healthy and feel beautiful during your treatments. You even get a free make-up kit.

Group support. Group support is where you'll meet people like you who are battling cancer. They had groups for people under 40, which worked nicely for me. These run once a week for 10 weeks. Listening to other people's challenges and sharing your own story definitely helps. It's nice to know you're not alone.

I met a patient in group support who had ovarian cancer. She told me that, when she got diagnosed, the first words to come out of her mouth were, "Why didn't I get breast cancer? Breasts are outside and can be removed easily." She told me doing a biopsy on an inner organ can be unbearable; it's something I never considered during my own plight.

Professional counselling. I ended up seeing a psychologist at Princess Margaret who works with post-treatment patients. I had thoughts about my husband's death that had not been dealt with. I was completely broken once my treatments were finished. My mind was so unclear and confused. I couldn't see any future. Counselling helped me get on with my life.

Mindfulness and meditation sessions. There were sessions at Princess Margaret for patients who had just finished their aggressive treatment. Those sessions were pretty helpful for me. They teach you how to forgive others and be positive in your life. They did mind exercises like body scans and focusing on all five senses. These exercises can help keep you calm and in control without worrying about the future. To me, it was self-reflection. It helped me learn more about myself.

Complementary therapies

Massage. Personally speaking, massage therapy gave me relief from ongoing pain, stress, and muscle tension. When my muscles get tense, I feel knots and so much stiffness. Deep-tissue massage with warm oil worked very well to relieve my stress. If your partner can do it, it's even better; you'll feel more connected and be more at ease in your own home.

NOTE: If you're going to get a professional massage, you'll be asked to provide a letter from your oncologist confirming it's safe for you to get a one.

Relaxation. Have some relaxation time each day. See yourself healing and coming out of the cancer. Be positive. Be happy. Practice deep breathing with some relaxing music or whatever makes you feel good.

Aqua therapy. Sitting in water helps a lot while your bones feel cracky and loose. Epsom salts can be calming. There were nights when I fell asleep in the tub because the soothing water took my pain away.

- Chapter 12 -
One Year Later

On September 13th, 2018, one year after I had my biopsy, I was at Women's College Hospital for an abdominal ultrasound. I was a walk-in patient and was told the walk-in wait time was about one to two hours. At about 10:30 AM the sonographer called my name and took me to a change room, providing me with the usual gown.

While doing the ultrasound, she found a cyst in my left ovary. Once she was done, she asked me to wait while she checked, to make sure the images were OK.

She came back 15 minutes later saying all was good, but that she needed to do some further imaging, through my vagina this time. That was a little uncomfortable. Once she was done, she left the room again to check the images. I waited. My thoughts started to cloud with fears of the cancer returning. She came back half an hour later and released me.

Right after that, I had an appointment with my psychologist, Chana, at Princess Margaret. I arrived at the 16th floor to see her, and was emotionally broken about the cyst.

Chana said she had never seen me this down before. "Where is your courage and your independent woman today?" she asked.

I told her I was giving up. It was getting too hard to cope with daily stuff. I was feeling lonely and depressed. I couldn't count on a single person for help—people have their own lives to deal with. My mood swings were out of control. One day I would be hyper, the next, totally down.

"I need help with my mood swings, Chana," I said. I was so tearful that day.

She advised me to plan a weekly schedule, where I made myself the top priority.

While still emotionally upset at the hospital, I called the assistant of my oncologist-gynecologist, Dr. Moulton, to see if he could see me to discuss the imaging I had done that morning. She found a cancellation at 4 PM and fit me in.

This is why Princess Margaret is my favourite. They are so quick and co-operative. Just to save a trip, time, and cost, they were willing to accommodate me. By 12 PM all the results were in my portal and there were no concerns, but I still felt it was worth talking to the doctor.

Dr. Moulton confirmed it was all good. I was OK.

- Chapter 13 -
Five Years Later

It took me five years to write this book. There were times when I would work on it full swing for four or five weeks, and then wouldn't do anything for the rest of the year. I was still dealing with emotions, pain, fatigue, and mood swings. The only difference was I had learned how to handle these things on a daily basis.

After five years, my periods started again, which made my GP worry. She sent me to do an ultrasound right away, as my uterus lining was so thickened. I was sent to a gynecologist for a biopsy. Same trauma and fear of reoccurrence. About three weeks later, the results came back and it was all clean. So, I was a little relieved.

Your body will have complications elsewhere. I had gall bladder stones for the past ten years; they didn't bother me much. But at the end of May, things changed. I was sent to an emergency room. I was kept there for three nights as a stone was stuck at the neck of a tube, causing a lot of inflammation and infection. I was kept on morphine and IV until surgery.

You must continue to self-advocate. Keep track of your body changes and keep checking them for any unusual changes. When you get a second chance to live, you don't want to waste it. Be positive, smile more, eat fresh, and be healthy

Self-advocacy. This book is about self-advocacy as much as my cancer journey. Self-advocacy is an ongoing process. If I have concerns about my body now, I don't hesitate to connect with my medical team and act. I am currently blessed to have a general practitioner who listens to me and never takes a chance.

Concentration. This was an ongoing issue after the treatment. I started to read more books, but I had a hard time focussing. I will read a book and forget its title. After five years it's getting better. Clarity is coming. I won't give up.

Aches and pains. Normal life has aches and pains. My best approach to them is to keep calm, do yoga, massage, regular walks, and eat properly. If you keep complaining about aches and pains, they won't go away—but the people who live with you will get tired of you. So be positive, and deal with it.

Fatigue. I still have good days and bad days. I feel more fatigue if I don't listen to my body when it tells me to stop. Or if I don't eat right. One thing I learned is my body is like a car: it must have supreme fuel for better performance.

Mood swings. Over the years since my diagnosis, I've really struggled with my moods. What I've learned is not to waste my energy on what isn't important, and to stay away from people who don't make me feel good. Pay attention to your surroundings. Step back from anything or anyone who is irritating you. Set boundaries. You are in charge of how you feel.

Memory. I still forget things easily and it still creates confusion. I still miss appointments if I haven't put a few alerts on. I forget words while having conversations. I forget the names of my favourite restaurants. I forget people's names a moment after we're introduced. It can be embarrassing if you are in a large group. Talk to your doctor if it's needed.

Conclusion

I hope this book, my experiences, and the step-by-step guides about what to expect help you in your journey. I hope this book gives you some courage to be your own advocate.

I've learned so much. I've learned to slow down. I've learned how important it is to have a supportive family. I've learned what true friends are. I've learned how we need to connect with those who have shared experience, so we can motivate and support each other.

Remember, you're still you; you're still that pretty face in the mirror; you're still strong.

Acknowledgements

I'm so grateful to acknowledge each and every staff member at Princess Margaret Cancer Centre in Toronto. They provided me with world-class medical treatment.

Thank you to Dr. Amir Eithan who has supported me throughout my treatment and provided me so much medical information about chemotherapy. He is the Executive Director of the Princess Margaret Cancer Centre Medical Oncology and Hematology Fellowship program and the Site Lead for Breast Medical Oncology. He also serves as the Cancer Care Ontario Systemic Therapy Lead for Toronto Central South and as the Vice-Chair of the Cancer Research Ethics Board at University Health Network.

Dr. Tulin Cil, Breast Surgical Oncologist at the University Health Network at Princess Margaret Cancer Centre.

Dr. Paaladinesh Thavendiranathan, who has shared his expertise to help put this book together. Dr. Thavendiranathan is a cardiologist at the Toronto General Hospital, University Health Network. He is the Director of the Ted Rogers Program in Cardiotoxicity Prevention which focuses on cardiac toxicity from systemic therapies including cancer therapy. He is also a Scientist at the Toronto General Hospital Research Institute (TGHRI).

Thank you to the lab staff, the sonographers, the triage nurses, my oncologists, my surgeon, and all the wonderful volunteers for helping me through this journey.

Thank you to my editor, Jan Robertson and my proofreader, David Balzer.

Special thanks to Dr. Shaliesh Gupta, Oncologist, Dr. Tanya Sehgal, Family Physician, Ruby Sahota MP, and to all my friends who have been there then and now, I love you all.

Be your own Advocate;
Own your Decisions;
Let the inner Power Heal.
- **Jag Kaur Takhar**

Manufactured by Amazon.ca
Bolton, ON

28359696R00050